THE *Skinny*
ACTIFRY
RECIPE BOOK

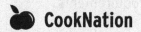
CookNation

The Skinny ActiFry Cookbook
Guilt-free & Delicious ActiFry Recipe Ideas:
Discover The Healthier Way to Fry!

A Bell & Mackenzie Publication
First published in 2014 by Bell & Mackenzie Publishing
Limited.
Copyright © Bell & Mackenzie Publishing 2014

ISBN 978-1-909855-34-2

A CIP catalogue record of this book is available from the
British Library

Disclaimer
This book is designed to provide information on the dishes
that can be cooked in the Tefal Actifry range only, results
and or timings may differ dependant on the product used.
Tefal UK were not involved in the recipe development or
testing of any of the dishes on this book.
Some recipes may contain nuts or traces of nuts. Those
suffering from any allergies associated with nuts should
avoid any recipes containing nuts or nut based oils.
This information is provided and sold with the knowledge
that the publisher and author do not offer any legal or
other professional advice.
In the case of a need for any such expertise consult with
the appropriate professional.
This book does not contain all information available on the
subject, and other sources of recipes are available.
This book has not been created to be specific to any
individual's or Tefal's requirements.

Credits:
Thank-you to Tefal UK for their kind permission to publish the Tefal ActiFry imagery in this book.

Contents

Contents

Contents

Introduction

Put simply the Tefal ActiFry is a fantastic new way of cooking that once discovered you won't be able to live without. This innovative and versatile appliance is a must for any modern kitchen and after you've tried it you won't look back! The ActiFry produces quick and easy healthy meals using a fraction of the oil required for traditional frying appliances. There is no preheating or mixing and it can cook a multitude of meals and snacks.....not just chips! Although having said that, chips are worthy of a special mention as the ActiFry produces some of the best crispy chips you will ever taste using a tiny amount of oil and therefore reducing quantities of fat.

How Does The Actifry Work?

A patented convection system moves hot air around the appliance in conjunction with a central paddle, which constantly stirs food ensuring even-cooking throughout. As the ActiFry requires no manual stirring or shaking it allows you to get on with other things while it cooks your perfect meal.

How Can It Produce Fried Food With So Little Oil?

The unique hot air system and paddle is so incredibly effective that there really is no need for vast quantities of oil to cook your food. One spoonful of oil is enough making it the healthiest way to fry.

Will Fried Food Taste Different Using The ActiFry?

If anything it will taste better than the fried food you are accustomed to eating. ActiFry has been designed to reduce the quantity of fat used in cooking without affecting the taste and whilst preserving flavour.

Cleaner, Safer, Healthier

The ActiFry requires only a spoonful of oil, which is around 100 times less than that used in a traditional deep fat fryer. Fresh oil is used each time you cook so there is no reusable oil creating strong odours and smoke – in fact the ActiFry is odourless. Using less oil is not only a healthier way to cook but also safer compared to traditional deep fat fryers. The ActiFry also pauses the cooking process when the lid is lifted allowing you to add ingredients or seasoning safely.

ActiFry Tips

Here are some useful hints and tips to get the best out of your ActiFry:

- When making chips don't make them too long as they can get broken by the paddle.
- Rinse the chips well before adding to the ActiFry to remove as much starch as possible.
- Thoroughly dry the chips before adding to the ActiFry to prevent any scorching.
- Remove your chips promptly when cooking process is complete to ensure they stay crispy.
- Clean your ActiFry after each use. All the parts easily come apart and are dishwasher safe.
- Do not use any abrasive materials or cleaning products as this can damage the non-stick coating.
- When cooking chips, don't add salt to the pan. Only add salt after they have been removed.
- When adding dried herbs and spices mix with a little oil or water first otherwise they can get blown around the pan by the convection system.
- Cut vegetables into small pieces to make sure they cook properly.
- Onions should be thinly sliced and separated.

- Read the manufacturers instructions. It sounds obvious but take some time to learn about all the functions of the ActiFry before using it. Not only will this make it easier and more fun to use but will also ensure you stay within the warranty terms and conditions should any problems with the appliance occur.

Our Recipes
In keeping with the effortless nature of the ActiFry, all our recipes are easy to follow with minimal preparation and cooking times. Recipes are divided into main meals, snacks and side dishes and each serves 4.

We use a wide variety of fresh and inexpensive ingredients, all of which can be sourced from your local supermarket. We've limited the need for too many one-off store cupboard ingredients which you are unlikely to use again and can be expensive.

While we recommend following the method for each of our recipes, we do encourage you to experiment with ingredients to suit your own taste, budget or according to what you have to hand in your kitchen. Don't be put off if you don't have one of the ingredients, try substituting with a different cut of meat, herb or spice. Cooking with the ActiFry should be enjoyable and the more you try new things, the more fun you will have.

We hope you enjoy *The Skinny ActiFry Cookbook*.

Skinny
ACTIFRY
CHICKEN
DISHES

Chicken Teriyaki & Noodles

Ingredients:

1 onion, sliced
2 tsp olive oil or sunflower oil
500g/1lb 2oz free range skinless chicken breast, sliced
1 tbsp water
2 carrots, cut into matchsticks
2 tbsp teriyaki sauce
250g/9oz precooked or 'straight to wok' cooked noodles
1 bunch spring onions/scallions, sliced lengthways into ribbons
Salt & pepper to taste

Method:

1. Place the onions & oil in the ActiFry and cook for 5 minutes.
2. Add the chicken, water, carrots & teriyaki sauce and cook for 14 minutes.
3. Add the noodles and cook for a further 2-4 minutes or until the chicken is cooked through and the noodles are piping hot.
4. Season and serve with the spring onion ribbons.

Teriyaki is a sweet Japanese sauce, which is widely available in most shops & supermarkets.

Spicy, Ginger Chicken Wings

Ingredients:

• Serves 4
• Cooking Time: 30-40 mins

3 red chillies, finely sliced
1 green pepper, sliced
1 tbsp freshly grated ginger
3 garlic cloves, peeled & finely sliced
1 tsp salt
1 tsp brown sugar
16 free range chicken wings
1 tsp olive oil or sunflower oil
Salt & pepper to taste

Method:

1. Place the chillies, peppers, ginger, garlic, salt & sugar in a food processor and pulse until blended.
2. Smother this blend over the chicken wings and leave to marinate for an hour or two (or longer if you like).
3. After this time place the chicken wings & oil in the ActiFry and cook for 30-40 minutes or until the chicken wings are cooked through and piping hot.
4. Season and serve.

If you have the time try marinating the chicken wings overnight before cooking.

Soy & Honey Drummers

Ingredients:

60ml/¼ cup soy sauce

2 tsp honey

2 garlic cloves

12 free range chicken drumsticks

1 tsp olive oil or sunflower oil

Lemon wedges to serve

Salt & pepper to taste

Method:

1. Place the soy sauce, honey & garlic in a food processor and pulse until blended.
2. Smother this blend over the chicken drumsticks and leave to marinate for an hour or two.
3. After this time place the drumsticks & oil in the ActiFry and cook for 30-35 minutes or until the chicken is cooked through and piping hot.
4. Season and serve with lemon wedges.

These drumsticks are great served with coleslaw and corn-on-the-cob.

Simple Crispy Fried Wings

Ingredients:

16 free range chicken wings
1 tsp garlic powder
½ tsp salt
1 tsp olive oil
Lemon wedges to serve
Salt & pepper to taste

• Serves 4
• Cooking Time: 30-35 mins

Method:

1. First rub the salt and garlic powder into the chicken wings.
2. Place the chicken & oil in the ActiFry and cook for 30-35 minutes or until the chicken is cooked through and piping hot.
3. Season and serve with lemon wedges.

A simple BBQ sauce makes a great addition to this recipe. You could add a tablespoon of sauce a couple of minutes before the end of cooking for an even glaze.

Chinese Chicken & Asparagus

Ingredients:

500g/1lb 2oz free range skinless chicken breast, cubed
1 tsp Chinese Five Spice powder
1 onion, sliced
200g/7oz asparagus tips, chopped
2 tsp olive oil or sunflower oil
3 tbsp chicken stock
2 Pak Choi/Bok Choy (Chinese cabbage) roughly chopped
250g/9oz precooked long grain rice
Salt & pepper to taste

Method:

1. First rub the 5 spice powder into the chicken pieces.
2. Place the onions, asparagus & oil in the ActiFry and cook for 5 minutes.
3. Add the chicken, stock & pak choi and cook for 12-14 minutes or until the chicken is cooked through.
4. Season and serve with the cooked rice.

You could serve this with extra soy sauce & a garnish of freshly chopped flat leaf parsley if you wish.

Mexican Chicken

Ingredients:

- Serves 4
- Cooking Time: 20-22 mins

1 red pepper, sliced
1 yellow pepper, sliced
1 red onion, sliced
2 tsp olive oil or sunflower oil
500g/1lb 2oz free range skinless
chicken breast, sliced
2 tbsp tomato paste/puree
200g/7oz ripe cherry tomatoes
1 tsp cayenne pepper
½ tsp cumin
1 tsp oregano or mixed herbs
½ tsp each salt & brown sugar
60ml/¼ cup chicken stock
Salt & pepper to taste

Method:

1. Place the peppers, onion & oil in the ActiFry and cook for 5 minutes.
2. Add the chicken, tomato puree, tomatoes, cayenne pepper, cumin, oregano, salt, sugar & stock and cook for a further 15-17 minutes or until the chicken is cooked through and piping hot.
3. Season and serve.

This is great served with tacos, sour cream and shredded lettuce.

Garlic & Basil Chicken

- Serves 4
- Cooking Time: 19-21 mins

Ingredients:

1 onion, sliced

2 garlic cloves, crushed

2 tsp olive oil or sunflower oil

400g/14oz free range skinless chicken breast, cubed

200g/7oz tinned chopped tomatoes

1 tbsp tomato puree/paste

½ tsp salt & brown sugar

4 tbsp freshly chopped basil

Salt & pepper to taste

Method:

1. Place the onions, garlic & oil in the ActiFry and cook for 5 minutes.
2. Add the chicken, tomatoes, puree, salt & sugar and cook for 12 minutes.
3. Sprinkle with the fresh basil, and cook for a further 2-4 minutes or until the chicken is cooked through and piping hot.
4. Season and serve.

Try serving with penne pasta and freshly grated Parmesan cheese.

Dry Rub Crispy Chicken Thighs

Ingredients:

- Serves 4
- Cooking Time: 30-40 mins

1 tsp garlic powder
½ tsp each cumin, salt, paprika, brown sugar & cayenne pepper
75g/3oz Parmesan cheese, grated
12 free range bone-in chicken thighs
2 tsp olive oil or sunflower oil
Salt & pepper to taste

Method:

1. Combine all the dry ingredients and grated cheese together.
2. Rub this mix into the chicken thighs.
3. Place the chicken wings & oil in the ActiFry and cook for 30-40 minutes or until the chicken thighs are cooked through, crispy and piping hot.
4. Season and serve.

You may like to leave out the cayenne pepper if you are serving this to young children.

Coriander Chicken

Ingredients:

500g/1lb 2oz free range skinless
chicken breast, cubed
2 tsp olive oil or sunflower oil
2 garlic cloves, finely sliced
1 tsp ground coriander/cilantro
½ tsp each ground cumin & salt
2 tbsp freshly chopped coriander/
cilantro
½ red onion, finely sliced
Salt & pepper to taste

Method:

1. Add all the ingredients to the Actify, except the chopped coriander and sliced red onion.
2. Cook for 12-14 minutes or until the chicken is cooked through.
3. Stir through the chopped coriander and sliced red onion.
4. Season and serve.

This dish can be served with rice or as a delicious pitta filling.

Coconut Cream & Peanut Chicken

Ingredients:

- Serves 4
- Cooking Time: 20-22 mins

2 garlic cloves, finely sliced
1 onion, sliced
2 tsp olive oil or sunflower oil
200g/7oz fresh chopped tomatoes
1 tbsp tomato puree/paste
75g/3oz peanuts, chopped
½ tsp each ground cumin, ginger & salt
1 tsp paprika
1 tbsp coconut cream
500g/1lb 2oz free range skinless chicken breast, cubed
2 tbsp freshly chopped flat leaf parsley
Salt & pepper to taste

Method:

1. Place the garlic, onions & oil in the ActiFry and cook for 5 minutes.
2. Add the tomatoes, puree, peanuts, cumin, ginger, salt, paprika & coconut cream and cook for 3 minutes.
3. Add the chicken and cook for a further 12-14 minutes or until the chicken is cooked through and piping hot.
4. Season, sprinkle with chopped parsley and serve.

Serve with cooked noodles and chopped peanuts to garnish if you wish.

Cashew & Citrus Chicken

Ingredients:

500g/1lb 2oz free range skinless chicken breast, cubed
1 tsp cornflour/cornstarch
2 garlic cloves, finely sliced
1 onion, sliced
2 tsp olive oil or sunflower oil
100g/3½oz cashew nuts, chopped
60ml/¼ cup orange juice
½ chicken stock/bouillon cube
2 tbsp freshly chopped coriander/cilantro
Salt & pepper to taste

Method:

1. Season the chicken & dust evenly with the corn flour.
2. Place the garlic, onions & oil in the ActiFry and cook for 5 minutes.
3. Add the cashew nuts & dusted chicken and cook for 8 minutes.
4. Add the orange juice & crumbled stock cube and cook for a further 5-7 minutes or until the chicken is cooked through and piping hot.
5. Season, sprinkle with chopped coriander and serve.

Dusting the chicken with flour should create a thick sauce.

Summer Corn Chicken

Ingredients:

- Serves 4
- Cooking Time: 23-25 mins

500g/1lb 2oz free range skinless
chicken breast, cubed
1 tsp cornflour/cornstarch
2 garlic cloves, finely sliced
1 red pepper, sliced
1 orange pepper, sliced
1 onion, sliced
1 tbsp water
2 tsp olive oil or sunflower oil
125g/4oz babycorn
125g/4oz carrots, sliced into batons
200g/7oz tinned creamed corn
Salt & pepper to taste

Method:

1. Season the chicken & dust evenly with the corn flour.
2. Place the garlic, sliced peppers, onions, water & oil in the ActiFry and cook for 5 minutes.
3. Add the mini corn cobs, carrots, creamed corn, stock & dusted chicken and cook for 18-20 minutes or until the chicken is cooked through and piping hot.
4. Season and serve.

This is a vibrantly coloured dish which makes a great summer recipe. Add a little water to the pan during cooking if needed.

Creamy Rosemary & Mushroom Chicken

Ingredients:

1 onion, sliced
200g/7oz mushrooms, sliced
2 tsp olive oil or sunflower oil
1 tsp fresh or dried rosemary, chopped
500g/1lb 2oz free range skinless chicken breast, cubed
200g/7oz tinned condensed mushroom or chicken soup
Salt & pepper to taste

Method:

1. Place the onions, mushrooms & oil in the ActiFry and cook for 5 minutes.
2. Add the rosemary & chicken & condensed soup and cook for 15-20 minutes or until the chicken is cooked through and the dish is piping hot.
3. Season and serve.

This recipe makes use of that great 'cheat' ingredient - condensed soup. Add a little water during cooking if needed.

Chicken & Spinach Kofta

Ingredients:

• Serves 4
• Cooking Time: 40 mins

500g/1lb 2oz free range chicken mince /ground chicken
2 garlic cloves, crushed
2 tbsp fresh breadcrumbs
½ tsp each ground turmeric, coriander/ cilantro, paprika, brown sugar & salt
400g/14oz potatoes, peeled & cubed
2 tsp olive oil or sunflower oil
200g/7oz spinach leaves
4 tbsp fat free Greek yoghurt
Lemon wedges to serve
Salt & pepper to taste

Method:

1. Put the chicken mince, garlic cloves, breadcrumbs, dried spices, sugar & salt in a food processor and pulse a few times until combined.
2. Take the mixture out and form into small meatballs with your hands.
3. Place the cubed potatoes in the ActiFry and cook for 15 minutes.
4. Add the chicken meatballs & and cook for a further 20 minutes or until the meatballs are cooked through.
5. Add the spinach and cook for 5 minutes or until the spinach begins to wilt.
6. Season and serve with a dollop of Greek yoghurt and lemon wedges.

If you don't have a food processor just use your hands to combine the meatball mixture.

Chicken Meatballs With Peppers

- Serves 4
- Cooking Time: 20-25 mins

Ingredients:

500g/1lb 2oz free range chicken mince/ground chicken
2 garlic cloves, crushed
2 tbsp fresh breadcrumbs
½ tsp each mixed herbs, paprika, brown sugar & salt
2 tsp olive oil or sunflower oil
3 large red or yellow peppers, sliced
400g/14oz tinned chopped tomatoes
2 tbsp tomato puree/paste
Salt & pepper to taste

Method:

1. Put the chicken mince, garlic cloves, breadcrumbs, mixed herbs, paprika, sugar & salt in a food processor and pulse a few times until combined.
2. Take the mixture out and form into small meatballs with your hands.
3. Place the meatballs and peppers in the ActiFry and cook for 10 minutes.
4. Add the chopped tomatoes & puree and cook for a further 10-15 minutes or until the meatballs are cooked through and piping hot.
5. Season and serve.

To make fresh breadcrumbs just whizz a slice of bread in the food processor for a few seconds.

Chicken & Almonds

Ingredients:

- Serves 4
- Cooking Time: 19-21 mins

2 garlic cloves, finely sliced
1 onion, sliced
2 tsp olive oil or sunflower oil
1 tbsp mild curry powder
½ tsp salt
1 tbsp tomato puree/paste
2 tbsp ground almonds
180ml/¾ cup tomato passata/sauce
500g/1lb 2oz free range skinless
chicken breast, cubed
3 tbsp low crème fraiche or fat free
Greek yoghurt
Salt & pepper to taste

Method:

1. Place the garlic, onions & oil in the ActiFry and cook for 5 minutes.
2. Add the curry powder, salt, tomato puree, almond, passata & chicken and cook for 14-16 minutes or until the chicken is cooked through and piping hot.
3. Season, stir through the crème fraiche and serve.

Serve with boiled rice and a chopped almond garnish if you wish.

Garlic Chicken

- Serves 4
- Cooking Time: 17-19 mins

Ingredients:

8 garlic cloves, finely sliced
2 onions, sliced
2 tsp olive oil or sunflower oil
½ tsp each of salt, cumin & turmeric
300g/11oz cherry tomatoes, halved
1 tbsp tomato puree/paste
500g/1lb 2oz free range skinless
chicken breast, cubed
2 tbsp freshly chopped flat leaf
parsley
Salt & pepper to taste

Method:

1. Place the garlic, onions & oil in the ActiFry and cook for 5 minutes.
2. Add the salt, cumin, turmeric, cherry tomatoes, tomato puree & chicken and cook for 12-14 minutes or until the chicken is cooked through and piping hot.
3. Season, stir through the chopped parsley and serve.

You could also use turkey breasts for this great low fat dish.

Chicken Fried Rice

Ingredients:

- Serves 4
- Cooking Time: 19-21 mins

1 onion, chopped
2 garlic cloves, crushed
125g/4oz peas
125g/4oz mushrooms, chopped
1 tbsp olive oil or sunflower oil
200g/7oz cooked chicken, chopped
or shredded
1 tsp Chinese Five Spice powder
500g/1lb 2oz precooked rice
2 free range eggs, beaten
1 tbsp soy sauce
2 tbsp freshly chopped flat leaf
parsley
Salt & pepper to taste

Method:

1. Place the onions, garlic, peas, mushrooms & oil in the ActiFry and cook for 12 minutes.
2. Add the chicken, 5 spice powder, rice, eggs & soy and cook for 7-9 minutes or until everything is cooked through and piping hot.
3. Season and serve with the chopped parsley sprinkled on top.

A handful of fresh beansprouts added to this recipe a few minutes before the end of cooking makes a good addition.

Skinny
ACTIFRY
MEAT
DISHES

Chinese Pork, Mushrooms & Cabbage

Ingredients:

1 onion, sliced
3 garlic cloves, crushed
2 carrots, cut into matchsticks
125g/4oz shitake mushrooms
2 tsp olive oil or sunflower oil
500g/1lb 2oz free range pork tenderloin, sliced into strips
2 Pak Choi/Bok Choy (Chinese cabbage), roughly chopped
1 tbsp soy sauce
2 tsp rice wine vinegar
1 bunch spring onions/scallions, sliced lengthways into ribbons
Salt & pepper to taste

Method:

1. Place the onions, garlic, carrots, mushrooms & oil in the ActiFry and cook for 5 minutes.
2. Add the pork, pak choi, soy sauce & rice wine vinegar and cook for 12-14 minutes or until the pork is cooked through.
3. Season and serve with the spring onion ribbons .

Pak choi is a Chinese cabbage readily available in most shops & supermarkets however it's fine to substitute for regular cabbage if you wish.

Spanish Fried Rice

Ingredients:

- Serves 4
- Cooking Time: 18-22 mins

2 red onions, chopped
2 garlic cloves, crushed
1 carrot, finely chopped
1 pepper, finely chopped
125g/4oz peas
125g/4oz chorizo, finely diced
2 tsp olive oil or sunflower oil
1 tsp paprika
1 tsp salt
500g/1lb 2oz precooked rice
2 free range eggs, beaten
2 tbsp water
2 tbsp freshly chopped flat leaf parsley
Salt & pepper to taste

Method:

1. Place the onions, garlic, carrots, peppers, peas, chorizo & oil in the ActiFry and cook for 10 minutes.
2. Add the paprika, salt, rice, eggs & water and cook for 8-12 minutes or until everything is cooked through and piping hot.
3. Season and serve with the chopped parsley sprinkled on top.

You could also add a little chopped chilli to this dish if you wish to give it a little more 'kick'.

Italian Beef & Beans

Ingredients:

1 onion, sliced
2 garlic cloves, crushed
2 tsp olive oil or sunflower oil
400g/14oz lean steak, sliced
400g/14oz tinned chopped tomatoes
400g/14oz tinned cannellini beans, drained
1 tbsp tomato puree/paste
1 tsp dried basil, oregano or mixed herbs
½ beef stock/bouillon cube
½ tsp brown sugar
2 tbsp freshly chopped flat leaf parsley
Salt & pepper to taste

Method:

1. Place the onions, garlic & oil in the ActiFry and cook for 5 minutes.
2. Add the sliced steak, chopped tomatoes, beans, tomato puree, dried herbs, crumbled stock cube & sugar and cook for 8-10 minutes or until everything is cooked through and piping hot.
3. Season and serve with the chopped parsley sprinkled on top.

Borlotti beans also make a good substitute for this dish.

The Classic Meat Sauce

Ingredients:

• Serves 4
• Cooking Time: 35-40 mins

1 onion, finely chopped
2 garlic cloves, crushed
2 carrots, finely chopped
2 tsp olive oil or sunflower oil
400g/14oz lean beef mince/ground beef
400g/14oz tinned chopped tomatoes
1 tbsp sundried tomato puree/paste
1 tsp dried thyme
½ beef stock/bouillon cube
½ tsp brown sugar
1 tbsp Worcestershire sauce/A1 steak sauce
Salt & pepper to taste

Method:

1. Place the onions, garlic, carrots & oil in the ActiFry and cook for 5 minutes.
2. Add the beef mince, chopped tomatoes, tomato puree, thyme, crumbled stock cube, sugar & Worcestershire sauce and cook for 30-35 minutes or until everything is cooked through and piping hot.
3. Season and serve.

This classic meat sauce is great served with spaghetti or sprinkled with cheese and served with tortilla chips.

Beef Kheema

- Serves 4
- Cooking Time: 30-40 mins

Ingredients:

1 onion, finely chopped
2 garlic cloves, crushed
2 tsp olive oil or sunflower oil
400g/14oz lean beef mince/ground beef
200g/7oz tinned chopped tomatoes
2 tbsp tomato puree/paste
1 tbsp medium curry powder
200g/7oz peas
½ beef stock/bouillon cube
½ tsp brown sugar & salt
2 tbsp freshly chopped coriander/cilantro
Salt & pepper to taste

Method:

1. Place the onions, garlic & oil in the ActiFry and cook for 5 minutes.
2. Add the mince, chopped tomatoes, tomato puree, curry powder, peas, crumbled stock cube, sugar & salt and cook for 25-35 minutes or until everything is cooked through and piping hot.
3. Season and serve with chopped coriander sprinkled over the top.

This should be a fairly dry Indian dish. Add a little water during cooking if required.

Cocoa Stir Fried Beef

Ingredients:

1 onion, sliced
2 red chillies, sliced
2 carrots, cut into matchsticks
2 red peppers, sliced
2 garlic cloves, crushed
2 tsp olive oil or sunflower oil
400g/14oz lean rump or sirloin steak, sliced
1 tbsp cocoa powder
2 tbsp tomato puree/paste
1 tbsp water
1 bunch spring onions/scallions, sliced lengthways into ribbons
Salt & pepper to taste

Method:

1. Place the onions, chillies, carrots, peppers, garlic & oil in the ActiFry and cook for 10 minutes.
2. Add the sliced steak, cocoa powder, puree & water and cook for 6-8 minutes or until everything is cooked through and piping hot.
3. Season and serve with the spring onions ribbons sprinkled on top.

This dish is great with served with rice or as the base to a simple crispy green salad.

Beef & Purple Sprouting Broccoli

- Serves 4
- Cooking Time: 16-18 mins

Ingredients:

1 onion, sliced
1 red chilli, sliced
3 garlic cloves, crushed
250g/9oz purple spouting broccoli/
broccolini roughly chopped
2 tsp olive oil or sunflower oil
400g/14oz lean rump or sirloin steak,
sliced
Salt & pepper to taste

Method:

1. Place the onions, chillies, garlic, broccoli & oil in the ActiFry and cook for 10 minutes.
2. Add the sliced steak and cook for 6-8 minutes or until everything is cooked through and piping hot.
3. Season and serve.

Purple sprouting broccoli is a gorgeous seasonal vegetable. This recipe works well with asparagus too.

Moroccan Lamb & Olives

Ingredients:

1 onion, sliced
2 tsp freshly grated ginger
2 garlic cloves, crushed
2 tsp olive oil or sunflower oil
2 handfuls black pitted olives, halved
400g/14oz lamb neck fillet, cut into strips
2 tsp cornflour/cornstarch
60ml/¼ cup lamb stock
½ tsp each ground nutmeg & cinnamon
2 tbsp freshly chopped coriander/cilantro
400g/14oz precooked long grain rice
Salt & pepper to taste

Method:

1. Place the onions, ginger, garlic & oil in the ActiFry and cook for 5 minutes.
2. Dust the lamb with cornflour and add to the ActiFry along with the stock & dry spices and cook for 18 minutes.
3. Add the cooked rice and chopped coriander and cook for a further 3-5 minutes or until everything is cooked through and piping hot.
4. Season and serve.

The nutmeg and cinnamon in this dish give it its North African aroma.

Greek Lamb Kebab

Ingredients:

1 tbsp dried oregano
4 tbsp olive oil
3 garlic cloves, crushed
3 tbsp red wine
Zest & juice of 1 lemon
600g/1lb 5oz lean lamb fillet, cut into 2cm/1 inch cubes
4 large pitta breads
4 tbsp fat free Greek yoghurt
1 baby gem lettuce shredded
Lemon wedges to serve
Salt & pepper to taste

Method:

1. Combine together the oregano, olive oil, garlic & red wine along with the juice and zest of 1 lemon in a large bowl.
2. Add cubed lamb, cover and leave to marinate for as long as possible, ideally overnight.
3. Remove the marinated meat from the bowl, place in the ActiFry and cook for 20-25 or until the lamb is cooked to your liking.
4. Serve the lamb in pittas with lettuce & yoghurt along with lemon wedges on the side.

You could add some crushed chilli flakes to this dish when serving if you wish.

Beef & Cheese Meatballs

Ingredients:

- Serves 4
- Cooking Time: 20-25 mins

500g/1lb 2oz lean beef mince / ground beef
1 garlic clove, crushed
2 tbsp fresh breadcrumbs
150g/5oz low fat cheddar cheese cut into 1cm/ ½ inch squares
2 tsp olive oil or sunflower oil
400g/14oz tomato passata/sauce
½ tsp each brown sugar & salt
2 tbsp tomato puree/paste
Salt & pepper to taste

Method:

1. Put the mince, garlic & breadcrumbs in a food processor and pulse a few times until combined.
2. Take the mixture out and form into small meatballs with your hands. Take a cube of cheese and push into the middle of each meatball and cover over with the meat to create a hidden cheese centre.
3. Place the meatballs in the ActiFry and cook for 15 minutes.
4. Add the tomato passata, salt, sugar & puree and cooked a further 5-10 minutes or until the meatballs are cooked through and the sauce is piping hot.
5. Season and serve.

This is great served with spaghetti. The cheese 'surprise' in the middle is always a big hit with the whole family.

Garlic Beef

Ingredients:

2 onions, sliced
8 garlic cloves, finely sliced
1 tbsp freshly grated ginger
2 tsp olive oil or vegetable oil
400g/14oz lean sirloin or rump steak, sliced
200g/7oz fresh beansprouts
Salt & pepper to taste

Method:

1. Place the onions, garlic, ginger & oil in the ActiFry and cook for 5 minutes.
2. Add the steak and cook for 4 minutes.
3. Add the beansprouts and cook for a further 2-3 minutes or until everything is cooked through and piping hot.
4. Season and serve.

Adjust the cooking time if you prefer your steak well done.

Sausage Gnocchi

Ingredients:

- Serves 4
- Cooking Time: 35 mins

8 pork or small Italian sausages
3 red or yellow peppers, sliced
1 onion, sliced
2 tsp olive oil or sunflower oil
800g/1¾lb premade gnocchi
Salt & pepper to taste

Method:

1. Place the peppers, onion & oil in the ActiFry and cook for 10 minutes. Remove from the ActiFry and put to one side.
2. Add the sausages & gnocchi to the ActiFry & cook for 20 minutes.
3. Remove the sausages and slice into 1cm thick discs.
4. Add the sliced sausages, sautéed peppers & onions to the gnocchi in the ActiFry and cook for a further 5 minutes or until the gnocchi is crispy on the outside and tender on the inside.
5. Season and serve.

Cooking the sausages before cutting makes them much easier to slice.

Mixed Beans, Beef & Rice

Ingredients:

• Serves 4
• Cooking Time: 18-20 mins

400g/14oz lean beef mince/ground beef
1 onion, sliced
2 garlic cloves, crushed
2 tsp olive oil or vegetable oil
120ml/½ cup tomato passata/sauce
400g/14oz tinned mixed beans, drained
1 tbsp tomato puree/paste
1 tsp dried rosemary or mixed herbs
½ beef stock/bouillon cube
½ tsp brown sugar
300g/11oz precooked long grain rice
1 tbsp fat free Greek yoghurt
2 tbsp freshly chopped flat leaf parsley
Salt & pepper to taste

Method:

1. Place the beef, onions & garlic in the ActiFry and cook for 5 minutes.
2. Add the tomato passatta, mixed beans, tomato puree, rosemary, crumbled stock cube & sugar and cook for 10 minutes.
3. Add the cooked rice and cook for a further 3-5 minutes or until everything is cooked through and piping hot.
4. Stir through the crème fraiche, season and serve with the chopped parsley sprinkled on top.

You could also serve this dish in taco shells or soft tortillas if you wish.

Pork & Apple Juice

Ingredients:

- Serves 4
- Cooking Time: 17-19 mins

2 onions, sliced
2 garlic cloves, crushed
2 carrots, cut into matchsticks
2 tsp olive oil or sunflower oil
500g/1lb 2oz free range pork
tenderloin, cut into strips
60ml/¼ cup pure apple juice
1 bunch spring onions/scallions,
sliced lengthways into ribbons
Salt & pepper to taste

Method:

1. Place the onions, garlic, carrots & oil in the ActiFry and cook for 5 minutes.
2. Add the pork & apple juice and cook for 12-14 minutes or until the pork is cooked through.
3. Season and serve with the spring onion ribbons.

Serve this dish with boiled rice, using all the juices out of the ActiFry to drizzle over the dish.

Thai Pork

Ingredients:

2 onions, sliced
2 garlic cloves, crushed
1 red pepper, sliced
2 carrots, cut into matchsticks
2 tsp olive oil or sunflower oil
500g/1lb 2oz free range pork
tenderloin, cut into strips
2 tbsp Thai red curry paste
1 tbsp water
300g/9oz precooked or 'straight to
wok' noodles
2 tbsp freshly chopped coriander/
cilantro
Salt & pepper to taste

Method:

1. Place the onions, garlic, peppers & carrots & oil in the ActiFry and cook for 5 minutes.
2. Add the pork, curry paste & water and cook for 10 minutes.
3. Add the cooked noodles and cook for a further 2-4 minutes or until everything is cooked through and piping hot.
4. Season and serve with the chopped coriander sprinkled over the top.

You could also use Thai green curry paste as an alternative.

Skinny
ACTIFRY
SEAFOOD
DISHES

Lightly Spiced Squid Rings

- Serves 4
- Cooking Time: 10-12 mins

Ingredients:

500g/1lb 2oz squid flesh cut into 1cm
/½inch wide rings
1 tsp paprika
½ tsp garlic powder
2 tsp olive oil or sunflower oil
Salt & pepper to taste

Method:

1. Pat dry the squid rings and coat with the paprika and garlic powder.
2. Place in the ActiFry with the olive oil and cook for 10-12 minutes or until crispy and cooked through.
3. Season and serve.

Fresh or frozen squid will work fine for this recipe.

Garlic & Spring Onion Prawns

Ingredients:

500g/1lb 2oz peeled king prawns/
jumbo shrimp
3 garlic cloves, peeled & thinly sliced
2 tsp olive oil or sunflower oil
A large bunch of spring onions/
scallions sliced
Salt & pepper to taste

- Serves 4
- Cooking Time: 13-15 mins

Method:

1. Pat dry the prawns and place in the ActiFry with the oil and sliced garlic. Cook for 10 minutes.
2. Add the chopped spring onions and cook for a further 3-5 minutes or until the prawns are pink and cooked through.
3. Season and serve.

Try serving with egg noodles and a little chopped chilli if you wish.

Salt & Pepper Prawns

- Serves 4
- Cooking Time: 13-15 mins

Ingredients:

500g/1lb 2oz peeled king prawns/
jumbo shrimp
1 tsp salt
1 tsp brown sugar
1 tsp ground black pepper
½ tsp Chinese Five spice powder
2 tsp olive oil or sunflower oil
1 red chilli, finely sliced
A small large bunch of spring onions/
scallions sliced lengthways

Method:

1. Pat dry the prawns and combine well with the salt, sugar, black pepper and Chinese five spice powder.
2. Place in the ActiFry with the oil and sliced chilli. Cook for 13-15 minutes or until the prawns are cooked through.
3. Sprinkle with sliced spring onions and serve.

Chinese five spice powder gives these prawns a distinctive taste which are lovely served with a fresh green salad.

Thai Curry Stir-Fry

Ingredients:

• Serves 4
• Cooking Time: 23-25 mins

1 onion, sliced
1 garlic clove, crushed
2 tsp olive oil or sunflower oil
1 carrot, cut into matchsticks
½ green pointed/Napa cabbage, shredded
1 red pepper, sliced
125g/4oz sugar snap peas
400g/14oz peeled king prawns/ jumbo shrimp
2 tbsp red Thai curry paste
200g/7oz fresh beansprouts
A large bunch of spring onions/ scallions sliced lengthways
Salt & pepper to taste

Method:

1. Place the onions, garlic & oil in the ActiFry and cook for 6 minutes.
2. Add the carrot, cabbage, peppers & peas and cook for a further 5 minutes.
3. Add the prawns, curry paste & beansprouts and cook for 12-14 minutes or until the prawns are cooked through.
4. Season & serve with the spring onions sprinkled over the top.

Freshly chopped coriander makes a good additional garnish to this tasty dish.

Peppers & Spinach Prawn Stir-Fry

Ingredients:

1 onion, sliced
2 garlic cloves, peeled & finely sliced
2 red peppers, sliced
2 tsp olive oil or sunflower oil
125g/4oz peas
400g/14oz peeled king prawns/
jumbo sgrimp
2 tbsp each water & soy sauce
1 tbsp Thai fish sauce
200g/7oz spinach leaves
300g/11oz precooked or 'straight to
wok' egg noodles
Lime wedges to serve
Salt & pepper to taste

Method:

1. Place the onions, garlic, peppers & oil in the ActiFry and cook for 4 minutes.
2. Add the prawns, peas & water and cook for a further 8 minutes.
3. Add the soy sauce, fish sauce, spinach & noodles and cook for 4-6 minutes or until the prawns are cooked through and the spinach & noodles are piping hot.
4. Season and serve with lime wedges.

Feel free to use a little more fish sauce to give additional savoury depth to this Thai dish.

Simple Sweet & Sour King Prawns

Ingredients:

- Serves 4
- Cooking Time: 16-18 mins

100g/3½oz tinned pineapple chunks
250ml/1 cup pineapple juice
1 onion, sliced
1 tbsp freshly grated ginger
½ red chilli, sliced
1 yellow pepper, sliced
2 tsp olive oil or sunflower oil
500g/1lb 2oz peeled king prawns/
jumbo shrimp
200g/7oz fresh beansprouts
400g/14oz precooked pilau rice
Salt & pepper to taste

Method:

1. First put the pineapple & juice in a food processor and blend to paste.
2. Place the onions, ginger, chilli, peppers & oil in the ActiFry and cook for 4 minutes.
3. Add the prawns and pineapple paste and cook for a further 10 minutes.
4. Add the beansprouts and cook for 2-4 minutes or until the prawns are cooked through and the beansprouts are piping hot.
5. Season and serve with the cooked pilau rice.

Traditional sweet & sour dishes often contain a little chilli, but feel free to leave it out if you prefer.

Spanish Butterfly Prawns

Ingredients:

2 onions, sliced
4 garlic cloves, peeled & finely sliced
1 red chilli, finely chopped
200g/7oz chorizo sausage, diced
2 tsp olive oil or sunflower oil
500g/1lb 2oz king prawns/jumbo shrimp, butterflied
4 soft tortilla wraps
2 baby gem/romaine lettuce, shredded
Lemon wedges to serve
Salt & pepper to taste

Method:

1. Place the onions, garlic, chilli, chorizo & oil in the ActiFry and cook for 4 minutes.
2. Add the butterflied prawns and cook for a further 10-12 minutes or until the prawns are cooked through and piping hot.
3. Season and serve with the tortilla wraps, shredded lettuce and lemon wedges.

To butterfly prawns: Leave the tail on. Work the knife into the length of the back of the prawn and push the meat apart without cutting fully open.

Scallops, Chorizo & Rice

Ingredients:

• Serves 4
• Cooking Time: 16-18 mins

1 onion, sliced
2 garlic cloves, crushed
200g/7oz chorizo sausage, finely sliced into discs
2 tsp olive oil or sunflower oil
200g/7oz peas
500g/1lb 2oz shelled & prepared scallops
400g/7oz precooked long grain rice
Lemon wedges to serve
Salt & pepper to taste

Method:

1. Place the onions, garlic, chorizo & oil in the ActiFry and cook for 4 minutes.
2. Add the peas and scallops and cook for a further 10 minutes.
3. Add the cooked rice and cook for a further 2-4 minutes or until the scallops are cooked through and the rice is piping hot.
4. Season and serve with lemon wedges.

Scallops are a delicious & relatively inexpensive shellfish. Use the freshest you can find to get the best taste.

Stir Fried Soft Shell Crab

- Serves 4
- Cooking Time: 14-16 mins

Ingredients:

1 onion, sliced
2 garlic cloves, peeled & finely sliced
2 red chillies, sliced
1 tbsp olive oil or sunflower oil
2 tbsp plain/all purpose flour
½ tsp each salt & sugar
12 small soft shell crabs
Salt & pepper to taste

Method:

1. Place the onions, garlic, chillies & oil in the ActiFry and cook for 4 minutes.
2. Mix together the flour, salt & sugar and use this to cover the crabs all over.
3. Add the floured crabs to ActiFry and cook for 10/12 minutes or until the crabs are cooked through and piping hot.
4. Season and serve.

Soft shell crabs are widely available at Chinese supermarkets.

Skinny
ACTIFRY
VEGETABLE DISHES

Balsamic & Rosemary Glazed Vegetables

Ingredients:

1 red pepper, sliced

1 red onion, sliced

1 carrot, cut into batons

200g/7oz whole button mushrooms

200g/7oz baby corn

200g/7oz spinach

2 tsp olive oil or sunflower oil

1 tbsp balsamic vinegar

1 tsp dried rosemary

Salt & pepper to taste

Method:

1. Place the vegetables, oil, balsamic vinegar & rosemary in the ActiFry.
2. Cook for 15-20 minutes or until the vegetables are tender.
3. Season and serve.

Fresh rosemary is fine to use too. Garnish with a little flat leaf parsley if you have it.

Tenderstem Broccoli & Anchovies

Ingredients:

600g/1lb 5oz tenderstem broccoli/
broccolini, sliced lengthways
1 onion, finely sliced
½ red chilli, finely chopped
5 tinned anchovy fillets in olive oil
(drain & reserve the oil)
Lemon wedges to serve
Salt & pepper to taste

- Serves 4
- Cooking Time: 15-20 mins

Method:

1. Place the broccoli in the ActiFry along with the onions, chilli, anchovy fillets and 1 tbsp of the reserved anchovy oil.
2. Cook for 15-20 minutes or until tender and cooked through.
3. Season and serve with the lemon wedges.

You could roughly chop the broccoli and toss with a little cooked rice to turn it into a main meal.

Creamy Pancetta & Sprouts

- Serves 4
- Cooking Time: 10-15 mins

Ingredients:

125g/4oz pancetta cubes
1 onion, finely sliced
500g/1lb 2oz Brussels sprouts, sliced
into thin discs
60ml/ ¼ cup vegetable stock or
water
60ml/ ¼ cup single cream/half & half
Salt & pepper to taste

Method:

1. Place the pancetta and onions in the ActiFry and cook for 5 minutes.
2. Add the sliced sprouts & stock and cook for a further 5-10 minutes or until tender and cooked through.
3. Stir through the single cream, season and serve.

Bacon and sprouts are a classic combination. This pancetta version adds an Italian twist.

Spicy Garlic & Lemon Kale

Ingredients:

- Serves 4
- Cooking Time: 15-20 mins

1 onion, finely sliced
1 tbsp olive oil or sunflower oil
250g/9oz kale, roughly chopped
2 tbsp water
½ tsp crushed chilli flakes
1 tbsp lemon juice
2 garlic cloves, crushed
Salt & pepper to taste

Method:

1. Place the onions and oil in the ActiFry and cook for 5 minutes.
2. Add the kale, water, chilli flakes, lemon juice & oil and cook for a further 10-15 minutes or until the kale is sautéed.
3. Season and serve.

Kale is packed full of vitamins and minerals and makes a great healthy side dish.

New Potatoes & Mustard Seed Spinach

Ingredients:

500g/1lb 2oz baby new potatoes, halved
1 garlic clove, crushed
1 tbsp mustard seeds
2 tsp olive oil or sunflower oil
200g/7oz spinach, roughly chopped
1 tbsp lemon juice
Salt & pepper to taste

Method:

1. Place the new potatoes, garlic, mustard seeds & oil in the ActiFry and cook for 20 minutes.
2. Add the spinach and lemon juice and cook for a further 10-20 minutes or until the potatoes are tender.
3. Season and serve.

If you can't source very small baby new potatoes slice larger potatoes rather than halving.

Fresh Ginger, Cabbage & Peas

Ingredients:

- Serves 4
- Cooking Time: 20-25 mins

1 onion, sliced
2 tsp olive oil or sunflower oil
1 tbsp freshly grated root ginger
1 garlic clove, crushed
1 green pointed/Napa cabbage shredded
250g/9oz peas
2 tbsp water
Salt & pepper to taste

Method:

1. Place the sliced onions, oil, grated ginger & garlic in the ActiFry and cook for 5 minutes.
2. Add the cabbage, peas & water and cook for a further 15-20 minutes or until the cabbage & peas are tender.
3. Season and serve.

If you use fresh peas rather than frozen peas you may need to add another tablespoon of water.

Crispy Honey Carrots

- Serves 4
- Cooking Time: 15-25 mins

Ingredients:

400g/14oz baby carrots, cut
lengthways
2 tsp olive oil or sunflower oil
2 tsp honey
Salt & pepper to taste

Method:

1. Place the carrots and oil in the ActiFry and cook for 15-25 minutes or until the carrots are crispy and tender.
2. Remove from the ActiFry and place in a bowl, drizzle with honey & combine well.
3. Season and serve immediately.

Use regular carrots cut into batons if you prefer.

Sweet Tomatoes, Asparagus & Spinach

Ingredients:

• Serves 4
• Cooking Time: 18-20 mins

400g/14oz cherry tomatoes, halved
½ tsp brown sugar
1 onion, sliced
2 tsp olive oil or sunflower oil
125g/4oz asparagus tips, roughly chopped
75g/3oz spinach
Salt & pepper to taste

Method:

1. Place the tomatoes, sugar, onions & oil in the ActiFry and cook for 10 minutes.
2. Add the asparagus tips and spinach and cook for a further 8-10 minutes or until tender and cooked through.
3. Season well and serve.

Ripe cherry tomatoes are great for this recipe but halved vine-ripened tomatoes will work well too.

Parmesan French Beans

Ingredients:

400g/14oz green beans
1 onion, sliced
1 tsp Worcestershire sauce/A1 steak sauce
2 tsp olive oil or sunflower oil
1 tbsp freshly grated Parmesan
Salt & pepper to taste

Method:

1. Place the French beans, onions, Worcestershire sauce & oil in the ActiFry and cook for 15-20 minutes or until tender and cooked through.
2. Sprinkle with the grated parmesan.
3. Season well and serve.

As an alternative use paprika rather than Worcestershire.

Crispy Turnip 'Fingers'

Ingredients:

2 white turnips, cut lengthways into 2cm/1inch wide 'fingers'
1 garlic clove, crushed
1 tsp mixed herbs
1 tsp paprika
2 tsp olive oil or sunflower oil
Salt & pepper to taste

- Serves 4
- Cooking Time: 20-30 mins

Method:

1. Pat dry the turnip 'fingers' and combine with the garlic, herbs, paprika and oil.
2. Place in the ActiFry and cook for 20-30 minutes or until the turnip is crisp on the outside & tender on the inside.
3. Season well and serve.

You could also try this recipe with celeriac.

Tapas Scrambled Omelette

Ingredients:

500g/11oz potatoes, peeled & cubed
½ red chilli, finely chopped
2 tsp olive oil
5 free range eggs, lightly beaten
2 tbsp freshly chopped flat leaf
parsley
Salt & pepper to taste

Method:

1. First rinse, then pat dry the potato cubes with kitchen towel.
2. Place in the ActiFry along with the chilli and oil. Cook for 30 minutes.
3. Add the eggs & parsley and cook for a further 5-10 minutes or until the potatoes are tender and the scrambled omelette is piping hot.
4. Season and serve.

Add some additional spice to this dish if you like.

Stir Fried Spring Greens

Ingredients:

- Serves 4
- Cooking Time: 15-20 mins

2 garlic cloves, crushed
1 red chilli, finely chopped
125g/4oz streaky bacon/side pork chopped
1 tsp olive oil or sunflower oil
400g/14oz shredded spring greens
2 tbsp water
Salt & pepper to taste

Method:

1. Place the garlic, chilli, bacon & oil in the ActiFry and cook for 5 minutes.
2. Add the Spring greens & water and cook for a further 10/15 minutes or until tender and cooked through.
3. Season well and serve.

Garlic and chilli work really well with fresh Spring greens. Discard any thick or tough stalks.

Aubergine & Capers

Ingredients:

2 aubergines/egg plants, cubed
2 handfuls pitted black olives, halved
2 tbsp chopped capers
1 tbsp lemon juice
2 tsp olive oil or sunflower oil
1 tbsp water
Salt & pepper to taste

Method:

1. Add all the ingredients to the ActiFry and cook for 15-20 minutes or until the aubergine is tender and cooked through.
2. Season well and serve.

You could serve this as the basis for a salad or tossed through linguine pasta with a little more olive oil.

Paprika Cauliflower

Ingredients:

1 onion, sliced
2 heads cauliflower, split into small florets
1 tsp paprika
½ tsp each garlic powder & salt
2 tsp olive oil or sunflower oil
Salt & pepper to taste

- Serves 4
- Cooking Time: 18-20 mins

Method:

1. Combine the florets together with the paprika, garlic & salt and place in the ActiFry along with the oil and onions.
2. Cook for 18-20 minutes or until the florets are tender and cooked through.
3. Season and serve.

Make sure the florets are small enough to cook quickly & evenly.

Sautéed Kale & Spinach

Ingredients:

1 onion, sliced
2 garlic cloves, crushed
400g/14oz shredded kale & spinach
1 tsp Worcestershire sauce/A1 steak sauce
2 tsp olive oil or sunflower oil
Salt & pepper to taste

Method:

1. Place the onion, garlic & oil in the ActiFry and cook for 4 minutes.
2. Add the Spring greens and Worcestershire sauce and cook for 10-12 minutes or until the Spring greens are tender.

If you are in a rush you can pick up bags of ready prepared shredded green vegetables in most supermarkets.

Herbed Butternut Squash

Ingredients:

2 butternut squash, peeled & cubed
2 tsp dried herbs
2 tsp olive oil or sunflower oil
Salt & pepper to taste

- Serves 4
- Cooking Time: 20-30 mins

Method:

1. Place the squash, herbs & oil in the ActiFry and cook for 20-30 minutes or until the cubes are crispy and tender.
2. Season and serve immediately.

You can use dried oregano or rosemary in place of mixed herbs.

Skinny
ACTIFRY
SIDE
DISHES

Homemade Shredded Tortilla Chips

Ingredients:

4 soft flour tortilla wraps
2 tsp olive oil or sunflower oil
½ tsp salt
Salt & pepper to taste

Method:

1. Roll the tortilla wraps and cut into thin shredded slices.
2. Place in the ActiFry with the oil and salt.
3. Cook for 8-11 minutes or until the shredded tortilla slices are crispy and golden.
4. Season and serve.

This makes a great finger-food snack or try serving as a side to a fresh tuna salad.

Cajun Fries

Ingredients:

800g/1¾lb potatoes
2 tsp olive oil or sunflower oil
2 tsp Cajun seasoning (Use shop
bought seasoning or make your own
version by combining ¼ tsp each of
brown sugar & salt along with ½ tsp
each of garlic powder, chilli powder
& ground cumin)
Salt & pepper to taste

- Serves 4
- Cooking Time: 28-32 min

Method:

1. Peel the potatoes and cut into thin fries. Give the fries a rinse and dry them off really well with kitchen towel.
2. Place the fries in the ActiFry along with the seasoning and oil.
3. Cook for 28-32 minutes or until the fries are crisp on the outside and tender on the inside.
4. Season and serve.

Use whichever type of potato you prefer. Desiree is a particularly versatile and tasty choice.

Indian Spiced Fries

Ingredients:

800g/1¾lb potatoes
2 tsp olive oil or sunflower oil
2 tsp medium curry powder (Use
shop bought curry powder or make
your own version by combining ¼ tsp
each of cayenne pepper & ground
coriander along with ½ tsp each of
garlic powder, turmeric & ground
cumin)
Salt & pepper to taste

Method:

1. Peel the potatoes and cut into thin fries. Give the fries a rinse and dry them off really well with kitchen towel.
2. Place the fries in the ActiFry along with the curry powder and oil.
3. Cook for 28-32 minutes or until the fries are crisp on the outside and tender on the inside.
4. Season and serve.

Use hot curry powder or a little more cayenne pepper in your mix if you prefer your fries to be spicier.

Bombay Potatoes

Ingredients:

800g/1¾lb potatoes
2 tsp olive oil or sunflower oil
½ tsp turmeric
½ tsp mustard seeds
1 tsp chilli powder
1 onion, sliced
Salt & pepper to taste

- Serves 4
- Cooking Time: 35-40 mins

Method:

1. Peel the potatoes and cut into small 2cm square cubes. Give the cubes a rinse and dry them off really well with kitchen towel.
2. Place in the ActiFry along with the spices and oil.
3. After 20 minutes of cooking add the sliced onion and continue to cook for a further 15-20 minutes or until the potato cubes and onions are tender.
4. Season and serve.

This crispy version of Bombay potatoes is ideal for ActiFry cooking.

Patatas Bravas

- Serves 4
- Cooking Time: 35-40 mins

Ingredients:

800g/1¾lb potatoes
2 tsp olive oil or sunflower oil
1 tsp paprika
2 tbsp low fat mayonnaise
1 garlic clove, crushed
Pinch of salt
Squeeze of lemon
Salt & pepper to taste

Method:

1. Peel the potatoes and cut into small 2cm square cubes. Give the cubes a good rinse and dry them off with kitchen towel.
2. Place in the ActiFry along with the paprika & oil.
3. Cook for 35-40 minutes or until the potato cubes are crispy on the outside and tender on the inside.
4. Meanwhile mix together the mayonnaise, garlic, salt & lemon to create a simple aiolo (garlic mayonnaise).
5. Season the potatoes and serve.

Patatas Bravas are a native Spanish dish often served with a spicy tomato sauce or, in this case, aiolo.

Fried Gnocchi

Ingredients:

800g/1¾lb premade gnocchi
2 tbp olive oil or sunflower oil
Salt & pepper to taste

- Serves 4
- Cooking Time: 20-30 mins

Method:

1. Place the gnocchi in the ActiFry along with the oil.
2. Cook for 20-30 minutes or until the gnocchi is crispy on the outside and tender on the inside.
3. Season and serve.

Gnocchi is traditionally boiled and served soft. This ActiFry version turns gnocchi into crisp golden dumplings which can be served as a quirky alternative to roast potatoes.

Sweet Potato Spicy 'Crisps'

- Serves 4
- Cooking Time: 15-20 mins

Ingredients:

3 large sweet potatoes
2 tsp olive oil or sunflower oil
½ tsp cayenne pepper or chilli powder
Salt & pepper to taste

Method:

1. Peel the potatoes and slice them thinly into 'crisps'.
2. Place in the ActiFry along with the cayenne pepper & oil and cook for 15-20 minutes or until they are cooked through and crispy.
3. Season and serve.

This is a great recipe which can be served as a snack or as a tasty side dish to a meal. Feel free to leave the potatoes unpeeled if you want a more rustic texture.

Mediterranean Potatoes

Ingredients:

- Serves 4
- Cooking Time: 35-40 mins

800g/1¾lb potatoes
2 tsp olive oil or sunflower oil
1 tsp dried basil/oregano or mixed herbs
1 garlic clove, crushed
25g/1oz sundried tomatoes, finely chopped
Lemon wedges to serve
Salt & pepper to taste

Method:

1. Peel the potatoes and cut into small 2cm square cubes. Give the cubes a good rinse and dry them off well with kitchen towel.
2. Place in the ActiFry along with the dried herbs, garlic & oil.
3. Cook for 20 minutes and add the finely chopped sundried tomatoes.
4. Cook for a further 15-20 minutes or until the potato cubes are crispy on the outside and tender on the inside.
5. Season and serve with lemon wedges.

You could also add some sliced sweet onions and halved cherry tomatoes to this recipe if you want a 'fresh' bite to this summery side dish.

Roast Porcini Potatoes

Ingredients:

800g/1¾lb potatoes
2 tsp olive oil or sunflower oil
25g/1oz dried porcini mushrooms
Salt & pepper to taste

Method:

1. Peel the potatoes and cut into small 2cm square cubes. Rinse, pat dry and put to one side.
2. Meanwhile place the dried porcini mushrooms in a food processor and whizz until they are turned into powder.
3. Mix the potatoes and porcini powder together and place in the ActiFry along with the oil.
4. Cook for 35-40 minutes or until the potato cubes are crispy on the outside and tender on the inside.
5. Season and serve.

Porcini mushrooms give a lovely depth of flavour to this simple potato side dish.

Luxury Fried Gnocchi

Ingredients:

800g/1¾lb premade gnochhi
2 tsp truffle infused olive oil
Salt & pepper to taste

- Serves 4
- Cooking Time: 20-30 mins

Method:

1. Place the gnocchi in the ActiFry along with the truffle oil.
2. Cook for 20-30 minutes or until the gnocchi is crispy on the outside and tender on the inside.
3. Season and serve.

Don't let the 'grand' title put you off making this super-easy side dish. Truffle oil is relatively inexpensive and can be bought at most supermarkets. It's really packed with flavour and adds a touch of luxury to the simplest of dishes.

Double Onions & Potatoes

Ingredients:

400g/14oz potatoes
400g/14oz sweet potatoes
2 tsp olive oil or sunflower oil
½ white onion, sliced
½ red onion, sliced
1 garlic clove, crushed
Salt & pepper to taste

Method:

1. Peel all the potatoes and cut into rough chunks. Give them a good rinse and dry well with kitchen towel.
2. Place in the ActiFry along with the oil.
3. Cook for 15 minutes and then add the onions & garlic.
4. Cook for a further 20-25 minutes or until the potatoes are crispy on the outside and tender on the inside.
5. Season and serve.

Using sweet potato and regular potatoes for this recipe gives this side dish a good counterbalance. Feel free to garnish with some freshly chopped herbs when serving.

Garlic & Olive Oil Ciabatta Croutons

Ingredients:

2 ciabatta rolls
2 tsp olive oil
2 garlic cloves, crushed

- Serves 4
- Cooking Time: 5-10 mins

Method:

1. Cut the ciabatta rolls into cubes and place in the ActiFry along with the oil and garlic.
2. Cook for 5-10 minutes until crispy & cooked.
3. Serve hot or cold.

Croutons make a great addition to soup and salads.

CONVERSION CHART: DRY INGREDIENTS

Metric	Imperial
7g	¼ oz
15g	½ oz
20g	¾ oz
25g	1 oz
40g	1½oz
50g	2oz
60g	2½oz
75g	3oz
100g	3½oz
125g	4oz
140g	4½oz
150g	5oz
165g	5½oz
175g	6oz
200g	7oz
225g	8oz
250g	9oz
275g	10oz
300g	11oz
350g	12oz
375g	13oz
400g	14oz

Metric	Imperial
425g	15oz
450g	1lb
500g	1lb 2oz
550g	1¼lb
600g	1lb 5oz
650g	1lb 7oz
675g	1½lb
700g	1lb 9oz
750g	1lb 11oz
800g	1¾lb
900g	2lb
1kg	2¼lb
1.1kg	2½lb
1.25kg	2¾lb
1.35kg	3lb
1.5kg	3lb 6oz
1.8kg	4lb
2kg	4½lb
2.25kg	5lb
2.5kg	5½lb
2.75kg	6lb

CONVERSION CHART: LIQUID MEASURES

Metric	Imperial	US
25ml	1fl oz	
60ml	2fl oz	¼ cup
75ml	2½ fl oz	
100ml	3½fl oz	
120ml	4fl oz	½ cup
150ml	5fl oz	
175ml	6fl oz	
200ml	7fl oz	
250ml	8½ fl oz	1 cup
300ml	10½ fl oz	
360ml	12½ fl oz	
400ml	14fl oz	
450ml	15½ fl oz	
600ml	1 pint	
750ml	1¼ pint	3 cups
1 litre	1½ pints	4 cups

Other COOKNATION TITLES

If you enjoyed 'The Skinny ActiFry Recipe Book' we'd really appreciate your feedback. Reviews help others decide if this is the right book for them so a moment of your time would be appreciated.

Thank you.

You may also be interested in other '**Skinny**' titles in the CookNation series. You can find all the following great titles by searching under '**CookNation**'.

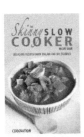

The Skinny Slow Cooker Recipe Book

Delicious Recipes Under 300, 400 And 500 Calories.

Paperback / eBook

More Skinny Slow Cooker Recipes

75 More Delicious Recipes Under 300, 400 & 500 Calories.

Paperback / eBook

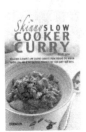

The Skinny Slow Cooker Curry Recipe Book

Low Calorie Curries From Around The World

Paperback / eBook

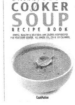

The Skinny Slow Cooker Soup Recipe Book

Simple, Healthy & Delicious Low Calorie Soup Recipes For Your Slow Cooker. All Under 100, 200 & 300 Calories.

Paperback / eBook

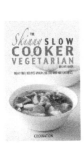

The Skinny Slow Cooker Vegetarian Recipe Book

40 Delicious Recipes Under 200, 300 And 400 Calories.

Paperback / eBook

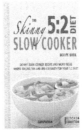

The Skinny 5:2 Slow Cooker Recipe Book

Skinny Slow Cooker Recipe And Menu Ideas Under 100, 200, 300 & 400 Calories For Your 5:2 Diet.

Paperback / eBook

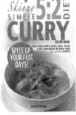

The Skinny 5:2 Curry Recipe Book

Spice Up Your Fast Days With Simple Low Calorie Curries, Snacks, Soups, Salads & Sides Under 200, 300 & 400 Calories

Paperback / eBook

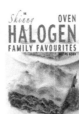

The Skinny Halogen Oven Family Favourites Recipe Book

Healthy, Low Calorie Family Meal-Time Halogen Oven Recipes Under 300, 400 and 500 Calories

Paperback / eBook

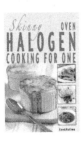

Skinny Halogen Oven Cooking For One

Single Serving, Healthy, Low Calorie Halogen Oven Recipes Under 200, 300 and 400 Calories

Paperback / eBook

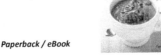

Skinny Winter Warmers Recipe Book

Soups, Stews, Casseroles & One Pot Meals Under 300, 400 & 500 Calories.

Paperback / eBook

The Skinny Soup Maker Recipe Book

Delicious Low Calorie, Healthy and Simple Soup Recipes Under 100, 200 and 300 Calories. Perfect For Any Diet and Weight Loss Plan.

Paperback / eBook

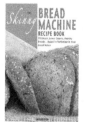

The Skinny Bread Machine Recipe Book

70 Simple, Lower Calorie, Healthy Breads...Baked To Perfection In Your Bread Maker.

Paperback / eBook

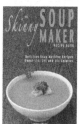

The Skinny Indian Takeaway Recipe Book

Authentic British Indian Restaurant Dishes Under 300, 400 And 500 Calories. The Secret To Low Calorie Indian Takeaway Food At Home

Paperback / eBook

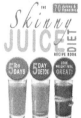

The Skinny Juice Diet Recipe Book

5lbs, 5 Days. The Ultimate Kick-Start Diet and Detox Plan to Lose Weight & Feel Great!

Paperback / eBook

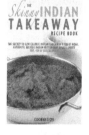

The Skinny 5:2 Diet Recipe Book Collection

All The 5:2 Fast Diet Recipes You'll Ever Need. All Under 100, 200, 300, 400 And 500 Calories

Available only on eBook

eBook

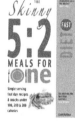

The Skinny 5:2 Fast Diet Meals For One

Single Serving Fast Day Recipes & Snacks Under 100, 200 & 300 Calories

Paperback / eBook

The Skinny 5:2 Fast Diet Vegetarian Meals For One

Single Serving Fast Day Recipes & Snacks Under 100, 200 & 300 Calories

Paperback / eBook

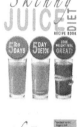

The Skinny 5:2 Fast Diet Family Favourites Recipe Book

Eat With All The Family On Your Diet Fasting Days

Paperback / eBook

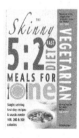

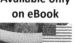

The Skinny 5:2 Fast Diet Family Favorites Recipe Book *U.S.A. EDITION*

Dine With All The Family On Your Diet Fasting Days

Available only on eBook

Paperback / eBook

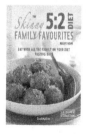

The Skinny 5:2 Diet Chicken Dishes Recipe Book

Delicious Low Calorie Chicken Dishes Under 300, 400 & 500 Calories

Paperback / eBook

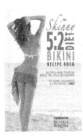

The Skinny 5:2 Bikini Diet Recipe Book

Recipes & Meal Planners Under 100, 200 & 300 Calories. Get Ready For Summer & Lose Weight...FAST!

Paperback / eBook

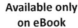

Available only on eBook

The Paleo Diet For Beginners Slow Cooker Recipe Book

Gluten Free, Everyday Essential Slow Cooker Paleo Recipes For Beginners

eBook

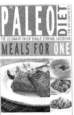

The Paleo Diet For Beginners Meals For One

The Ultimate Paleo Single Serving Cookbook

Paperback / eBook

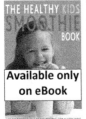

The Paleo Diet For Beginners Holidays

Thanksgiving, Christmas & New Year Paleo Friendly Recipes

Available only on eBook

eBook

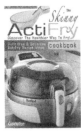

The Healthy Kids Smoothie Book

40 Delicious Goodness In A Glass Recipes for Happy Kids.

Available only on eBook

eBook

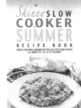
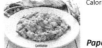

The Skinny Slow Cooker Summer Recipe Book

Fresh & Seasonal Summer Recipes For Your Slow Cooker. All Under 300, 400 And 500 Calories.

Paperback / eBook

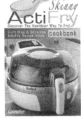

The Skinny ActiFry Cookbook

Guilt-free and Delicious ActiFry Recipe Ideas: Discover The Healthier Way to Fry!

Paperback / eBook

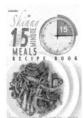

The Skinny 15 Minute Meals Recipe Book

Delicious, Nutritious & Super-Fast Meals in 15 Minutes Or Less. All Under 300, 400 & 500 Calories.

Paperback / eBook

The Skinny Mediterranean Recipe Book

Simple, Healthy & Delicious Low Calorie Mediterranean Diet Dishes. All Under 200, 300 & 400 Calories.

Paperback / eBook

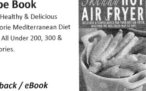

The Skinny Hot Air Fryer Cookbook

Delicious & Simple Meals For Your Hot Air Fryer: Discover The Healthier Way To Fry.

Paperback / eBook

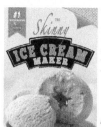

The Skinny Ice Cream Maker

Delicious Lower Fat, Lower Calorie Ice Cream, Frozen Yogurt & Sorbet Recipes For Your Ice Cream Maker

Paperback / eBook

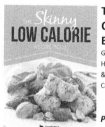

The Skinny Low Calorie Recipe Book

Great Tasting, Simple & Healthy Meals Under 300, 400 & 500 Calories. Perfect For Any Calorie Controlled Diet.

Paperback / eBook

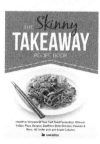

The Skinny Takeaway Recipe Book

Healthier Versions Of Your Fast Food Favourites: Chinese, Indian, Pizza, Burgers, Southern Style Chicken, Mexican & More. All Under 300, 400 & 500 Calories

Paperback / eBook

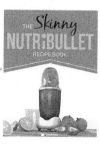

The Skinny Nutribullet Recipe Book

80+ Delicious & Nutritious Healthy Smoothie Recipes. Burn Fat, Lose Weight and Feel Great!

Paperback / eBook

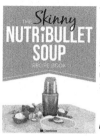

The Skinny Nutribullet Soup Recipe Book

Delicious, Quick & Easy, Single Serving Soups & Pasta Sauces For Your Nutribullet. All Under 100, 200, 300 & 400 Calories.

Paperback / eBook

Made in the USA
Middletown, DE
03 December 2019